Creating a Healthier You

ONE DAY AT A TIME

30 HEALTHY HABITS TO GET YOU MOVING, EATING BETTER & FEELING BETTER

• • •

BY EVERY SUNRISE PRESS

© Every Sunrise Press

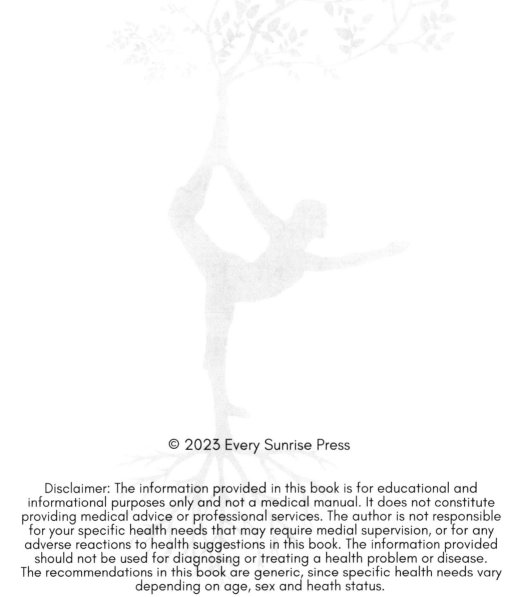

© 2023 Every Sunrise Press

Disclaimer: The information provided in this book is for educational and informational purposes only and not a medical manual. It does not constitute providing medical advice or professional services. The author is not responsible for your specific health needs that may require medial supervision, or for any adverse reactions to health suggestions in this book. The information provided should not be used for diagnosing or treating a health problem or disease. The recommendations in this book are generic, since specific health needs vary depending on age, sex and heath status.

Welcome to 30 days of resetting some habits to build a better lifestyle.

This book will offer 30 suggestions to get you started on a new healthy path. Many want to lose weight and feel great quickly, but building the habits that will keep you going and keep the weight off and feeling great for years to come is the goal!

Every day a new habit will be added. Make it to the end of 30 days and you will have changed 30 habits to create a healthier lifestyle!

● ● ●

Use the Healthy Habit Swap Pages to write the day you make the switch and which habit you chose. Add a check mark to the square at the top of each habit once you have tried it at least once!

Each swap has a section for notes!

Let's get started!

HEALTHY HABITS

PAGE

1-3	HEALTHY HABITS SWAP
4	DRINK HALF YOUR WEIGHT IN WATER
5	ADD 1X 15 MINUTE WALK
6	PAUSE THE SOCIAL MEDIA
7	ADD 10-15 MINUTES OF STRETCHING EACH EVENING
8	STRETCH ROUTINE EXAMPLE
9	REMOVE POP AND SUGAR FILLED BEVERAGES
10	SPEND TIME WITH FAMILY, FRIENDS AND LOVED ONES
11	ADD 10 MINUTES OF FULL MORNING SUNLIGHT TO YOUR ROUTINE
12	PLAN ONE WEEK OF MEALS
13-14	MEAL PREPARTION
15	START JOURNALING
16	START THE DAY WITH 8-10 MINUTES OF SKIPPING OR REBOUNDING
17	INCREASE YOUR VEGETABLE INTAKE
18	SWAP YOUR OILS
19	PICK UP A PHYSICAL BOOK AND READ
20	DITCH THE FABRIC SOFTENER & DRYER SHEETS

HEALTHY HABITS

PAGE	
21	FINISHED DINNER? STOP EATING!
22	PICK SOMETHING YOU LOVE AND DO IT FOR FUN!
23	LET'S TRY TO BREAK-FAST A LITTLE LATER TODAY.
24	EAT THREE FRUITS A DAY
25	TURN OFF THE TECHNOLOGY ONE HOUR BEFORE GOING TO SLEEP
26	ENJOY SWEETS? LET'S MAKE SOME SWAPS!
27	TRY FOR TWO 25 MINUTE WALKS/HIKES EACH WEEK
28	EPSOM SALT BATHS
29	REMOVE ALCOHOL FOR ONE WEEK STARTING TODAY
30	STOP AND BREATHE!
31	START PLANKING
32	MAKE TIME FOR NATURE
33	LEMON WATER IN THE MORNING…BEFORE YOUR MORNING COFFEE
34	DRY BRUSHING
35	WRITE DOWN YOUR GOALS
36	GET 6-7 HOURS OF QUALITY SLEEP, WITH 2-3 BEFORE MIDNIGHT

HEALTHY HABIT SWAP

DATE   **HEALTHY HABIT**

HEALTHY HABIT SWAP

DATE   **HEALTHY HABIT**

_____   _____

_____   _____

_____   _____

_____   _____

_____   _____

_____   _____

_____   _____

_____   _____

_____   _____

_____   _____

_____   _____

HEALTHY HABIT SWAP

DATE   **HEALTHY HABIT**

----------   --------------------

----------   --------------------

----------   --------------------

----------   --------------------

----------   --------------------

----------   --------------------

----------   --------------------

----------   --------------------

----------   --------------------

----------   --------------------

DRINK HALF YOUR WEIGHT IN WATER

Essential for life, water is necessary for our physical and mental functions. We can only last a few days without water. Our body is made of approximately 55% (women) or 60% (men) water.

BENEFITS

- Helps flush toxins
- Helps give you energy
- Helps with weight loss goals
- Helps in digestion
- Allows brain to focus and function
- Aids in clear plump skin
- Helps boost immune system function
- Delivers oxygen throughout your body
- Helps lubricate joints
- Helps maintain blood pressure

BEVERAGES TO BOOST YOUR WATER INTAKE

The following beverages are some of the beverages included in your water intake:
Pure water, herbal tea, sparkling water, lemon water

_____ LBS (CURRENT WEIGHT)/2 = _____ OUNCES

NOTES:

ADD 1x 15 MINUTE WALK ☐

Walking is another benefit to your physical and mental health. Can you add a short walk in today? It can be around the block a few times, on a treadmill, around the mall or even up and down the stairs in your home.
Have you ever tried a forest walk? Forest bathing allows your body to decrease anxiety, inhale the benefits of the trees and bring a calm all while giving you energy.

BENEFITS
- Improve your heart health
- Improve muscle tone and joint lubrication
- Improve sleep
- Boost immune function
- Increase energy
- Help calm anxiety/stress
- Increase brain function
- Increase circulation
- Help digestion

CHALLENGE
Get your shoes/boots/sandals on and hit the sidewalk, forest trails, playground loop or mall.

NOTES:

PAUSE THE SOCIAL MEDIA

Did you think we meant forever? NO! Try not to look at social media accounts for the first one to two hours after waking up. How about waiting until you are done your entire morning routine?

BENEFITS

- Keeps your mind clearer and more focused
- You can jump into your tasks more efficiently
- More focus on you and your family
- Your morning routine will be more effective
- Decrease anxiety from things you read or saw
- Increase connection with people in real life
- You do not start your day comparing yourself to others
- Once you start to scroll, you can be on there for a very long time

CHALLENGE

Other than important calls/texts/etc set your phone aside and do not keep it in your hand as you prepare for your day.

NOTES:

ADD 10-15 MINUTES OF STRETCHING EACH EVENING

This sounds like the last thing you may want to do before bed, right? This is an easy one to sneak in. Why not try to stretch when watching your favorite show? Or set a timer for 10 minutes, and don't look at it, and just start to stretch. The time will go by so fast!

BENEFITS
- Helps calm your body and mind to prepare you for sleep
- Improves your sleep quality
- Removes tension from your muscles
- Helps circulation
- Increases range of motion
- Improves posture
- Decreases negative stress response in our body
- Helps decrease tension headaches

CHALLENGE
Have your mat or area ready, set an alarm on your phone to stretch before bed. Have a family? Make it a family stretch.

NOTES:

STRETCH ROUTINE EXAMPLE
30 seconds to 1 minute per stretch repeat 3 times

Rag Doll Stretch

Feet hip width apart, toes forward, inhale and hinge forward from the hips with a flat back. Cross your arms and hold the opposite elbow. Have a slight bend to the knee and hang. Do not forget to breathe!

Downward Dog

Kneel on your mat with your spread hands under your shoulders Tuck your toes under and breathe out and activate your abs as you push your body off the mat. Your body will be in an inverted V shape. Press your hands and feet into the floor. Make sure your neck is relaxed and keep breathing.

Sumo Squat Stretch

Stand tall with feet separate enough to do a deep squat. Take a breath and squat with a flat back. Remain in a deep squat for as long as possible.

Bear Hug

Wrap your arms around the back of your shoulders in a hug position, tuck your chin to your chest and bend forward. Remember to breathe.

Nose to Ceiling

Turn your face to the left then lift your nose to the ceiling facing forward breathe and then end on the right side. Trace an arc with your nose. Repeat 10 times each way. Left to right then right to left.

Door Frame Stretch

Place your arms in a 90 degree L with hands facing the ceiling. Place both arms at opposite sides of a door frame, lean in and breathe.

Child's Pose

Spread your knees as wide as your mat and let your belly rest between your thighs. Place forehead on the floor and breathe.

REMOVE POP AND SUGAR FILLED BEVERAGES

These "oh so sweet" (including diet versions) beverages may be your desired thirst quenchers or craving satisfiers, but they are not helping keep your body hydrated or healthy! Why not replace this with some lemon water sweetened with 1 tsp of maple syrup or honey?

DANGERS

- The sugar turns into fat in your liver
- Erodes your tooth enamel
- Significantly increases belly fat
- There is no nutritional value, you are drinking empty calories that cause damage to your body
- They are addictive! Sugar is the only thing humans are born addicted to!
- Increase your risk of heart disease
- Increase your risk of cancer
- Very irritating for your stomach, causing heartburn or acid reflux

THE SWITCH

Lemon water with honey or maple syrup
Sparkling water
Water infused with berries and mint
Fresh juiced vegetables

NOTES:

SPEND TIME WITH FAMILY, FRIENDS AND LOVED ONES

Do you find you are always so busy and never have a second left in the day? This can be tiresome and lead to burnout. We need to take time to spend with people we enjoy to be around.

BENEFITS
- A constant support system
- You can share experience with them
- Provides a sense of belonging
- Increases your endorphins
- Helps you see your self-worth
- Helps you stay balanced and on a healthy track
- Decreases anxiety and depression

MAKING SOME PLANS
Plan a family brunch or dinner
Go on a hike
Go on a trip
Camp
Plan a game night

NOTES:

ADD 10 MINUTES OF FULL MORNING SUNLIGHT TO YOUR ROUTINE

Most of us are stuck indoors and do not see any sun until we are out the door running to work or school. We should all try to get in some morning sun within the first 1 - 1.5 hours after waking!

This is especially beneficial in winter as the sun is further away and harder to get, especially in the Northern Hemisphere.

BENEFITS

- Helps reset our circadian rhythm (body clock) to help you sleep better at night
- Boost your mood
- Lower stress
- Decrease seasonal affective disorder (SAD)
- Help with skin ailments
- Provides that much needed vitamin D that helps our body fight off disease and viruses
- Helps with weight management
- Increases metabolsim

GET THAT SUNLIGHT

Open the blinds during your morning routine
Eat breakfast outside
Sunglasses off during your morning commute
Use a Seasonal Affective Disorder (SAD) Lamp on those gloomy days

NOTES:

PLAN ONE WEEK OF MEALS

Planning meals helps save time, energy, calories and stress!
Planning your meals in advance allows you to be in control.

BENEFITS
- You will not waste money on take out or waste too many ingredients building a last minute meal
- This saves time! You know exactly what you will make each day.
- This will keep the calories in check helping with your weight
- Minimize food waste as you will know exactly what you have in your stock and will use it during your week.
- HEALTHIER EATING! When you get hungry, you tend to eat whatever you can, this way you will plan ahead and eat what is on your healthy menu.

CHALLENGE
Set up your meal plan on the same day each week prior to going grocery shopping.

NOTES:

MEAL PREPARATION

MONDAY
BREAKFAST

LUNCH

DINNER

SNACK

TUESDAY
BREAKFAST

LUNCH

DINNER

SNACK

WEDNESDAY
BREAKFAST

LUNCH

DINNER

SNACK

THURSDAY
BREAKFAST

LUNCH

DINNER

SNACK

MEAL PREPARATION

FRIDAY
BREAKFAST

LUNCH

DINNER

SNACK

SATURDAY
BREAKFAST

LUNCH

DINNER

SNACK

SUNDAY
BREAKFAST

LUNCH

DINNER

SNACK

NOTES

START JOURNALING

Our minds are like a full filing cabinet of the good, the bad, the to-do lists, the stressors, the must do's, the dreams, the urgent matters and not so urgent matters. Journaling daily is a way to help ease the stress our mind has on a daily basis.

BENEFITS

- Helps reduces stress
- Declutter your brain
- Help with depression
- Help you find patterns in your day to day that can cause stress and plan strategies to change it
- Helps you sleep better and more sound
- Organize the files in your brain
- Increase creativity
- Regulates emotions
- Help you stay in control of your emotions

JOURNAL AWAY

Grab a notebook at home or a specific journaling book and start today. A few short minutes a day is all you need!

NOTES:

START THE DAY WITH 8-10 MINUTES OF SKIPPING OR REBOUNDING

Did you enjoy jumping on a trampoline when you were younger? Do you still like it now? With a few minutes a day, you can start the day off right!

BENEFITS

- Jump start your metabolism first thing on the morning
- Strengthens you heart
- Decreasing inflammation throughout your body
- Helps with lymphatic drainage, which is important in flushing toxins and stagnation from your body
- Tightens every part of your body with every jump
- Boost your mood
- Help with weight loss goals
- Protects joints form chronic fatigue
- Activates the pituitary gland, stimulating bones.
- Boosts your G-Force, strengthening the musculoskeletal system

BOUNCING GOALS

Wake up, wash up and make your way to your rebounder or start those jumping jacks. Notice the energy burst you feel at the end and how activated your muscles feel!

NOTES:

INCREASE YOUR VEGETABLE INTAKE

Do you remember your mom or dad says, remember to eat your vegetables? They didn't say that for fun! It is so beneficial for a healthy body.

BENEFITS

- Lowers blood pressure
- May help prevent disease/cancer
- Aids in better digestion
- Keeps blood sugar levels stable
- Decrease inflammation in the body due to antioxidant levels
- Helps us reach our daily fiber intake requirements
- Helps keeps moisture in our skin
- Helps keep our brain sharp
- Helps boost your immune system

VEGETABLE GOALS

Try and eat the Rainbow!
Red, Orange, Yellow, Green, Purple
TIP: Make extra so you have one or two vegetable prepared for the next day.

NOTES:

SWAP YOUR OILS

Canola oil, grape-seed oil, sunflower seed oil, soybean oil are all oils we should try to avoid. These have only in recent decades been added to our foods and diets, leading to chronic inflammation, fatigue, autoimmune issues, heart disease, cancer and nutrient deficiencies.

BENEFITS OF EXTRA VIRGIN OLIVE OIL, COCONUT OIL, AND AVOCADO OIL

- Reduces chronic inflammation
- Lower blood pressure
- High in antioxidants
- High in oleic acid (fatty acid) which can have a positive effect on cancer cells
- Reduces the risk of stroke
- Beneficial for brain health
- Aids in bone health
- Antibacterial properties

OIL SWAP

Use avocado oil or coconut oil to cook at high temperatures.
Use extra virgin olive oil for dressing and cooking at low temperatures.

NOTES:

PICK UP A PHYSICAL BOOK AND READ

Who doesn't love a good book? Life has become so busy, we simply don't have time to just sit and read but it is definitely something we should do!
After dinner, before bed, after you put the kids to sleep, grab a book and read one page, one chapter, 10 minutes, or one hour.

BENEFITS

- Helps to increase your vocabulary
- Stimulates your brain aiding in a healthier body
- Decrease cognitive decline
- Helps expand your imagination and creativity
- Learn different facts
- Expand your thinking patterns
- Helps you focus
- Another form of entertainment that doesn't include technology
- Help improve writing skills
- Reduce stress

BOOK PLANNING

Everyone likes a good show, why not watch a bit of your show then turn it off to end your evening with book reading. It relaxes your eyes, mind and will help you sleep better!

NOTES:

DITCH THE FABRIC SOFTENER & DRYER SHEETS

Everyone loves fresh smelling laundry! Fabric softener & dryer sheets provides soft fresh smelling clothing that keeps your clothing feeling like new for longer. These have been proven to cause a burden on your health.

DANGERS OF FABRIC SOFTENER

- Can cause allergies
- Can cause skin irritations
- Can cause dermatitis
- Can cause difficulty breathing
- Can damage your reproductive health
- Trigger asthma
- Toxic for our water sources
- Some colors linked to cancer
- Cause severe stress on your nervous system

ALTERNATIVES

Fabric Softener
White Vinegar with 4-5 drops of organic lavender essential oil

Dryer Sheets
100% Wool Dryer Balls

NOTES:

FINISHED DINNER? STOP EATING!

Who doesn't like a snack or something sweet after dinner? One of the best way to control what you eat and keep the calories down is through keeping your dinner as your last food intake of the day!

BENEFITS
- Gives your body time to digest before bed
- May help burn your fat cells for energy
- Aids in better sleep
- Allows your body to focus on regeneration while asleep
- Reduces your chances of over eating

WHAT TO HAVE AFTER DINNER
Focus on non-caloric beverages like water, warm water with lemon, herbal teas.

NOTES:

PICK SOMETHING YOU LOVE AND DO IT FOR FUN!

Do you love gardening? Sewing? Do you want to learn a new skill? Take some time out of your week to learn something new, do something new, or get back into something you love!

BENEFITS
- Improves confidence
- Improves creativity
- Build a memory base
- Reduce stress
- Improve focus
- Learn a new skill or master a skill
- Provides a new meaning for you!

SET SOME MINI GOALS FOR SUCCESS

Start by researching what you are interested in. Narrow in on what you'd like to learn.
Get the necessary tools & start! Youtube, how-to books, quick web searches can give you quick tutorials to start right and with confidence.

NOTES:

LET'S TRY TO BREAK-FAST A LITTLE LATER TODAY.

Waking up in the morning, many of us can not wait to eat, but should we?

BENEFITS
- Generally helps reduce your caloric intake
- Increases weight loss
- Improve metabolic health
- Reduce inflammation in the body
- Reduce oxidative stress
- Increase cell repair due to the body focusing on your cells and repairing instead of digesting your food

CHALLENGE
Can you push back breakfast even one hour.

NOTES:

EAT THREE FRUITS A DAY

There are so many delicious and nutritious fruits available, each has so many benefits to our bodies.

BENEFITS

- High in fibre
- High in water – helps hydrate our cells
- Provides beneficial vitamins and minerals for our eyes, organs and skin
- Aids in digestive regularity
- Many fruits are high in antioxidants
- Reduces inflammation
- Many have antibacterial properties

ADD SOME FRUITS

LEMONS – High in vitamin C, antioxidants, antibacterial, anti-cancerous, thiamin, potassium, folate, vitamin A

APPLES – High in fibre, boost heart health and weight loss, high levels of quercetin, potassium, calcium

BLUBERRIES – Contains anthocyanin, an antioxidant protecting against heart disease, cancer, stroke. They contain pterostilbene, preventing plaque on the arteries

Have fun with fruit. Try some you've never had and be sure to get at least 3 in each day.

NOTES:

TURN OFF THE TECHNOLOGY ONE HOUR BEFORE GOING TO SLEEP

This is tough. We all look at our phones, want to watch a movie to relax or finish up some work before bed. But this is causing some major stress on our bodies.

BENEFITS
- Increases the production of melatonin making it easier to fall asleep
- It is easier for your mind to calm and get ready for bed
- Blue light on our phone or TV makes our body think it's daytime/daylight, creating an alertness in our bodies

CHALLENGE
Put down the phone, shut off the TV and pick up a journal and write or pick up a book and read.

NOTES:

ENJOY SWEETS? LET'S MAKE SOME SWAPS!

The only thing we are born craving is sugar. It's difficult to think about removing sugar. Sugar hides in so many items we buy too!

DANGERS OF PROCESSED SUGAR CONSUMPTION

- Increases blood pressure
- Makes insulin and blood sugar spike
- Aids in weight gain
- Significantly increases belly fat
- Aids in diabetes
- Increased risk of heart attack and strokes
- Increase your risk of heart disease
- Increase your risk of cancer
- Develops cavities in teeth
- Damages your skin cells
- Your cells repair process is slowed
- Sugar turns into fat in our body

CHALLENGE

Make some switches! Maple syrup, dates, and coconut sugar are all better options for your sweets. Find your favorite cookie recipe and make a large batch substituting the sweetener. Freeze them so you always have a healthier treat available. Just don't eat too many at a time!

NOTES:

TRY FOR TWO 25 MINUTE WALKS/HIKES EACH WEEK

You heard this one before right? You know all the benefits of walking and spending time in the forest. Now let's rev up your cardio game!

BENEFITS

- Boosts your immune systems several times a week
- Breathe in clean air to help expand your lungs
- Increases your ability to stay active longer
- Stronger muscles and bones
- Aids in heart health
- The sounds you hear in nature helps to reduce stress
- Increases your ability to problem solve
- Increases your attention span
- It is easier on your joints

CHALLENGE

Pick two days this week to go on this walk. Find a friend or family member to walk with you or have an audio book or 25 minute playlist of your favorite songs ready to listen to. You will not regret a walk once you have completed it

NOTES:

EPSOM SALT BATHS

Epsom salts added to warm bath water is quite soothing and has so many health benefits. Epsom salts are made up of magnesium, sulfur and oxygen, and while you are soaking in the bath, they infuse into your skin, cells and organs.

BENEFITS
- Boosts magnesium in your body
- Positive effects on your heart
- Helps calm the nervous system
- Helps promote sleep
- Reduce stress reactions
- Aids in constipation
- Helps with muscle recovery
- Aids in pain
- Calm inflammation

CHALLENGE
Set out two times this month to prepare a bath and soak in the benefits of the Epsom salts. You can add some lavender or chamomile to add to the relaxation.

NOTES:

REMOVE ALCOHOL FOR ONE WEEK STARTING TODAY

Removing alcohol or cutting down your consumption can be the best thing you do for your health! Alcohol aids in inflammation, immunity issues, heart issues, and diseases.

BENEFITS

- Aids in weight loss
- Skin appears clearer and more vibrant
- More energy
- Reduces inflammation
- Aids in a stronger immune system
- Improves mental health
- Decreases chances of a fatty liver
- Decreases heartburn and stomach upset due to the acidity

CHALLENGE

Pick a non-alcoholic beverage to substitute your alcoholic beverages for one week. Notice how your body feels without alcohol.

NOTES:

STOP AND BREATHE!

We all breathe, but do we breathe properly? Our bodies keep going because we breathe. We breathe approximately 22,000 time a day. Breathing allows oxygen to enter our bloodstream and all our organis. It allows us to function.

BENEFITS OF FOCUSED BREATHING

- Decreases anxiety
- Expands your lungs
- Decreases muscle tension
- Adds oxygen to your blood
- Aids in focus
- Boosts immune system
- Boosts energy
- Boosts circulation
- Helps control the nervous system
- Aids in digestion

CHALLENGE

Get in a comfortable position laying down or sitting in a chair. Relax, close your eyes and loosen your neck and shoulders. Take slow deep breaths in from your nose, fill out your diaphragm like you are opening an umbrella and blow out from your mouth as if you are blowing out into a juice straw. Picture closing the umbrella as you are blowing out.
Try to do this 3 minutes a day!

NOTES:

START PLANKING

Planking is when you hold your body in a flat straight line with your hands to elbows on the floor and your toes curled under to keep your body hovering over the floor. Doing a plank strengthens your transverse abdominis, rectus abdominiis, obliques and glutes.

BENEFITS

- Strengthens your entire body. Each plank you tighten every part of your body
- Strengthens your core muscles and back muscles, which is important to keep your back strong.
- Decreases your chances of injury doing strenuous activities
- Aids in elongating your back and neck.
- Improves flexibility
- Boosts energy
- Improves balance

CHALLENGE

Place your body in a flat position and put yourself on your elbows and toes. The first day hold the position for as long as possible. Put a timer on and see how long you can hold it. Every day add five seconds to your previous plank. Before you know it you will be doing one, two, or five minute planks!

NOTES:

MAKE TIME FOR NATURE

Have you every heard of forest bathing? Walking in nature to clear your mind? Grounding to balance your body? They're all of great benefit!

BENEFITS

- Decreases anxiety levels
- Creates a calm on your body
- Decreases irritability
- Decreases cortisol (stress hormone)
- Enjoy the beautiful scenery, sounds, and animals.
- Increases your ability to focus
- Aids in grounding your body

CHALLENGE

Set time and put it in your calendar to get outdoors. In the winter, you can sled or cross country ski. In the summer, pack a picnic and hike in your nearest conservation area.

NOTES:

LEMON WATER IN THE MORNING...BEFORE YOUR MORNING COFFEE

Start your day off right with some cleansing, energizing lemon water. There are so many benefits and it will help start your day off right!

BENEFITS
- A whole foods vitamin C
- Water Intake Increase
- Decreases coffee cravings
- Packed with other beneficial vitamins
- Clearer skin
- Aids in digestion
- Our body needs the ionic & trace minerals
- Increases hydration & electrolytes

RECIPE
1 Whole Freshly Squeezed Lemon
20-30 Drops Trace Minerals
1-2 TSP Celtic Sea Salt
1/4 TSP Ground Cinnamon Spice
Topped with Warm Filtered Water

NOTES:

DRY BRUSHING

Let's help detox!
Dry brushing is an exfoliation of the skin while it gently massages your skin.
It's best to do before showering.
Use firm strokes, without damaging your skin, and start at your feet and moving upwards towards your heart in long circular motions. Start with feet, then shin/ankle, followed by thigh/hamstring/buttocks, then belly and back then chest and neck. Be sure to always move towards your heart.

BENEFITS

- Removes dead skin
- Helps boost your circulation
- Helps with lymphatic drainage
- Helps fill in your skin
- Helps flow blood to areas with stagnation
- Aids in digestion

CHALLENGE

Get a dry brush and start with 2 minutes of dry brushing before a shower or bath.

NOTES:

WRITE DOWN YOUR GOALS

Writing is something we do not seem to do anymore. All the techonology has us texting and typing but not about our goals. Be descriptive, get them down on digital or physical paper.

BENEFITS

- Provides motivation when you see it written down
- Makes you accountable
- Goals seem more achievable
- Vividly writing it down is strongly correlated with goal success
- Have something tangible you can look back on to help keep your goal real!

GOALS
GOAL 1

GOAL 2

NOTES:

GET 6-7 HOURS OF QUALITY SLEEP, WITH 2-3 BEFORE MIDNIGHT

Sleep, why sleep? There are so many things I need to get done in a day! You can be more efficient by getting enough sleep! The 30 Days of a healthier you can help you sleep better!

BENEFITS
- Better sleep quailty
- More energy upon waking
- Boosts your immune system
- Helps increase memory function
- Decreases anxiety
- Decreases risks of diseases
- Helps with weight control
- Healthier heart
- More amicable
- Easier to get along with
- Regulates blood sugar

SLEEPING GOALS
Tonight try to go to bed 30 minutes early. Each night following add another 30 minutes until you are sleeping at 9 or 10PM

NOTES:

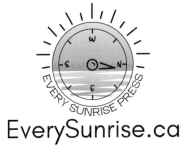